The Alana Marie Project Presents

The Heaviest Tear: Grieving Couples

Tony & Nicole Campbell

Wayne & Kelsey Hambrick

Ryan & Ashley Lehart

Marcus & Tondrea Maclin

Antwon & Marquisse Watson

Curtis & Amanda Winkle

BK
ROYSTON
Publishing

BK Royston Publishing
http://www.bkroystonpublishing.com
bkroystonpublishing@gmail.com

© 2024

Cover Design: Elite Cover Designs

ISBN-13: 978-1-963136-60-9

Printed in the United States of America

Dedication

To the Couples:

Tony & Nicole Campbell,

Wayne & Kelsey Hambrick, Ryan & Ashley Lehart,

Marcus & Tondrea Maclin, Curtis & Amanda Winkle

Thank you all; thank you for your, "yes!" Each of you entered our lives at different times—some before grief, and some after—but all of you have left a lasting mark on our hearts. When we asked you to be part of this book and share intimate details about your loss, you agreed without hesitation. We understand writing your story takes a lot out of you. It's as if you relive the experiences all over again. Thank you for believing in us and trusting us with such a personal part of your life. Thank you for pouring out your heart with words to offer hope and encouragement to other couples. May this book be the start of something bigger and greater than we could have ever imagined!

With heartfelt gratitude,

Antwon & Marquisse Watson

Table of Contents

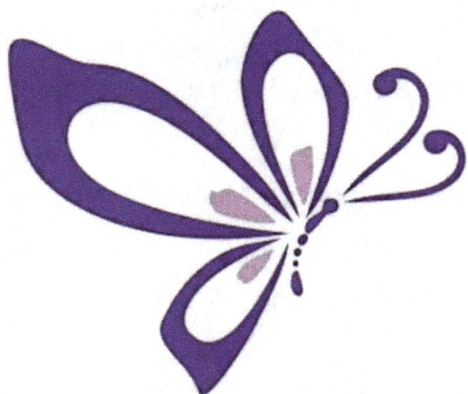

Introduction

In 2014, we began our journey as grieving parents. Being in a relationship comes with its own set of challenges, and losing a baby adds a new level of complexity to that. Since we started our grief journey, we've seen many relationships and marriages end after the loss of a child. Grief can allow couples to either grow together or drift apart. Sadly, we've witnessed the latter far too often. Grief changes who you are both as an individual and as a couple. It can make you feel misunderstood, especially when the other partner isn't open about their own grief.

When we envisioned the idea for this book, many people already knew what we faced together as a couple. However, we wanted to give other couples a chance to share how grief has affected their relationships. Our goal is to elevate our mission of encouragement, empowerment, and support. We pray any couple reading this book will connect with the shared stories to find hope and peace.

To the couples navigating the difficult journey of losing a child, we see you. The path won't be easy, but it will eventually lead you to peace. Commit to growing closer through your grief rather than letting it drive you apart. Fight for your relationship. We are here, cheering you on every step of the way!

Antwon & Marquisse Watson

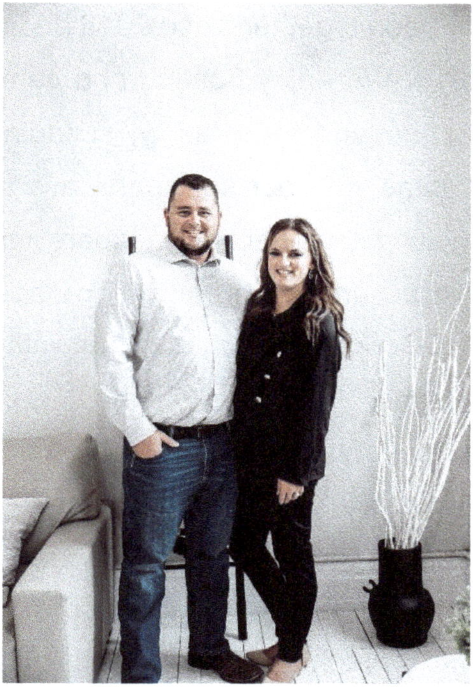

Tony & Nicole Campbell

There is no silence louder than a room where a doctor is attempting to find your baby's heartbeat.

We have been together since 2015 and married since 2018. We enjoy boating and camping at Lake Cumberland as a family, spending quiet time at home with our son, and have recently began golfing together in our spare time. We also have a nonprofit organization called "The Hayden & Crue Project" that we run with Kelsey and Wayne Hambrick who are also collaborators on this book.

We had just celebrated one year of marriage in April of 2019, and in May we found out we were going to be parents for the first time. The beginning of the pregnancy was easy, with minimal complications. However, after I entered the second trimester, several complications arose. One of them was excessive bleeding, which is usually indicative of a miscarriage. When the bleeding didn't subside, we made several urgent doctors' visits. However, despite the bleeding, the baby appeared to be healthy. At sixteen weeks, even though we were nervous about our pregnancy, we decided to go to Becoming Mom in Mason, OH to determine the gender of our baby. It was there where we learned we were having a girl. That day, we decided her name would be Hayden Rae Campbell. Unfortunately, a little over two weeks later, we received some of the most devastating news we would ever receive.

On the morning of August 31st, 2019, we had a gut feeling something was seriously wrong with Hayden. Call it a parent's intuition, but something was telling us to check her heartbeat on our fetal doppler, even though we had found a strong heartbeat the night before. After spending what felt like hours attempting to find Hayden's heartbeat and remaining unsuccessful, we decided to give it some time and go furniture shopping for a dresser for her nursery. Throughout the entire shopping experience, there was a heaviness both of us felt as we tried to believe everything would be okay. After purchasing a dresser and coming home, we attempted to find Hayden's heartbeat yet again, but we were just as unsuccessful as we were before. At that point, we called our best friend, Kelsey Hambrick, who has a background in nursing. She was with her sister, Bailey Schwartz, who at the time was a labor and delivery nurse. They both agreed we should come over so they could help us find Hayden. After both made an attempt to find Hayden, they agreed I should go to the hospital just to be sure.

They said Hayden was still small, and it was possible she was hiding. Even though our friends were trying to be positive, we knew, at that moment, something was horribly wrong.

The seven-minute drive to the hospital felt like a lifetime as we checked into triage on the Labor and Delivery floor. After a nurse's failed attempt at finding a heartbeat, a doctor with a mobile ultrasound came in. As the doctor attempted to find the heartbeat of our daughter, the silence in the room was deafening. Minutes felt like hours, and as soon as the doctor returned the wand to its position, it was confirmed we had officially lost her. I was being admitted to labor and delivery and would be induced to give birth to our daughter, who would be born sleeping. After nineteen stressful hours, Hayden Rae Campbell was born, weighing 137 grams; she was seven and a half inches long. We had no idea the journey the grief of losing our daughter would take us on, but nearly five years later, we are still actively dealing with the waves of grief that now exist permanently in our lives.

The days, weeks, months, and even years after our loss have been difficult, and that's putting it lightly. The doctors cleared us to start trying for another baby in October 2019, and that tested our relationship in a way we hadn't expected. We were left with more questions than answers as to why there were complications in our first pregnancy, which left both of us nervous about entering another pregnancy if there was an increased chance of losing another baby. However, after the loss, we both grieved differently. That resulted in us having differing opinions concerning when we should try to have another baby or if we should even try at all. We argued more frequently than we ever had during the past. We also began to understand why, statistically, there are many couples whose marriages do not survive after that kind of loss. We saw a therapist together a few times, but we both determined we didn't feel that route was the right path for us. Over time, we decided to speak to a therapist individually, which was extremely beneficial in helping us each handle our individual triggers and grief.

Five months after losing Hayden, we found out we were having another baby. As excited as we were, we knew, no matter what, we were going to be extremely nervous during the entire pregnancy. The true feeling of excitement for a pregnancy was stolen from us after our loss, and no amount of time gives us that back. We were both constantly waiting for something to go wrong, and when similar complications arose during our second pregnancy, we were convinced we were going to experience another loss.

Our constant hoping and praying led us to meeting our amazing son on September 29th, 2020, just a little over a year after the worst day of our lives. We still experience grief in waves, especially when we have to explain to our son he has a sister, whom he unfortunately won't get to meet during this lifetime. We talk about Hayden as often as we can and even went on to start a nonprofit with our friends, Kelsey and Wayne Hambrick, who also experienced the loss of their son three months after we lost Hayden. The Hayden & Crue Project develops Angel Suites, which provides families the time and space to be with their babies in the hospital before saying their final goodbyes. That project has helped us grow and heal after our loss, knowing our daughter, while she is not here with us, is leaving behind her legacy. Hayden's name, along with Crue's, has allowed us to reach out and connect with so many families who have experienced losing a child. As much as those families have thanked us for our help, they don't realize they are also helping us navigate our loss and our grief.

There is no easy to way to continue surviving after experiencing the loss of a child. It is a common misconception time heals all wounds; we have not found that to be the case. There is no amount of time that will allow us to completely heal from losing Hayden. However, our grief and our coping tactics have changed. In the beginning, there were so many days when we thought we would never feel happy again. As time goes on, we find our days of crippling grief and pain are fewer and farther between, but they are still there. Grief usually creeps up on us when we least expect it. Some sudden triggers include: reading a book or watching a movie with the main character being named Hayden, attending a baby shower for a little girl, and seeing pictures of milestones for children who are the same age Hayden should be. There are also more obvious things, such as the anniversary of losing her and her birthday. We used to feel guilty when our grief would set in at events such as a baby shower or a birthday party, but over time, we have learned that is normal and nothing for which we need to apologize. It is okay for some days to be worse than others, and it is okay to feel happy again. Giving ourselves grace to unapologetically feel our emotions after our loss has been a tough lesson to learn, but it has also helped us tremendously during the hard days. Unfortunately, there is no manual to help us navigate loss, and there isn't anyone on this Earth who grieves the same way. It is always important to remember you can lean on the people around you, ask for help when you need it, and understand your grief won't ever fully go away, but the weight of the loss won't be suffocating forever. Finally, it is always acceptable to talk about your child and the loss you experienced. Don't be concerned with making other people uncomfortable; the world deserves to know your child, no matter how fleeting their life was.

"Knowing you were gone before you arrived broke me. Birth and death should never collide. No parent should have to say goodbye before they've even said hello." – Sara Millen

To learn more about The Hayden &
Crue Project visit:

http://www.thehaydenandcrueproject.com/

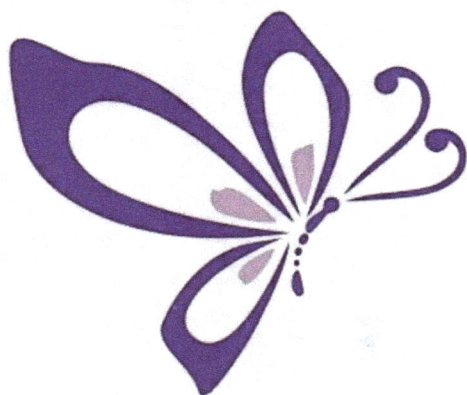

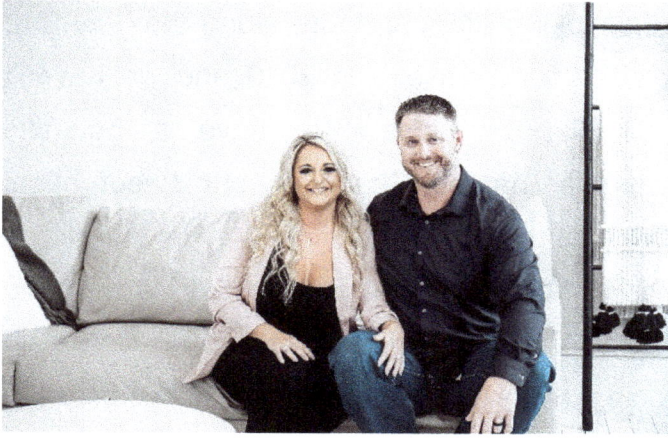

Wayne & Kelsey Hambrick

Just Keep Swimming

There is not a day that goes by when we don't
replay every detail of the day when we lost
you, our sweet baby boy, our biggest lesson,
and our brightest blessing.

After taking many detours along the way, our paths finally crossed in 2019 and we haven't looked back since. We have a beautiful daughter named Charleigh, our sweet angel Crue, and our vibrant rainbow after the storm, Oliver. We are co-founders of the Hayden and Crue Project, which places "Angel suites" in local hospitals and helps bring a little comfort to families going through unimaginable loss. When we aren't working or running the kids all over town, we enjoy spending our time at the lake, getting together with friends and family, and soaking up all the "chill" nights we can get in at home!

As a couple, our relationship was in hyper speed from the start. After both of us had been in many failed relationships, we were happy and excited to begin our future. Shortly after, we learned we had a baby on the way; they would be our first joint child to join our blended family. We decided to name our baby boy Crue. For the first nineteen weeks, our pregnancy was nothing out of the ordinary. It wasn't until after the twentieth week when we noticed some of the symptoms we were experiencing were not typical. We were often battling swelling, high blood pressures, and headaches.

We started seeing a maternal fetal medicine doctor for the hypertensive episodes and the continued swelling. Our team of doctors often had the conversation with us it wasn't "if" we developed preeclampsia, it was "when." On Friday, December 6th, at just 24 weeks pregnant, we were seen at our high-risk clinic and it was decided that we would stay in the hospital for continued monitoring due to hypertensive readings that would not subside with interventions that could take place in the office. Our hope of a short, overnight stay quickly turned into something far more serious in the blink of an eye.

Before we knew it, we were receiving steroid injections for Crue's lungs, and the doctor prescribed magnesium to help prevent seizures brought on by the high blood pressures. Shortly after, they transferred us to a hospital with higher level of care capability.

After countless tests, imaging, and examinations, the doctors concluded the preeclampsia had become severe enough to cause brain swelling, and we decided to move forward with an emergency C-section. As a mother, having your husband and the doctors make the decision to deliver your baby in order to save your own life is an incredibly tough pill to swallow. Despite the desperate pleas to the doctors to give our baby more time, we knew the pregnancy had to end; Crue needed to be delivered in order for him to have a chance to thrive.

At 4:11 p.m. on Monday, December 9, 2019, we gave birth to a crying, perfect little boy weighing one pound and sixteen ounces; he was twelve point five inches long. That crying was music to our ears. His eyes weren't open yet. His little fingers and toes were so long, and his facial features reminded us so much of his big sister, Charleigh. We were overwhelmed with love. Crue was so tiny, but yet so strong, and we were ready to fight his NICU journey alongside him.

On Wednesday, December 11th, the doctors called us to meet with them. That was not a normal thing, and we knew it. They informed us Crue had suffered bilateral grade 4 brain bleeds. We knew the possible outcome was grim, but we weren't ready to give up on our son. We decided to cling onto faith and continue to be Crue's biggest cheerleaders.

Over the course of the next few days, Crue was a little rock star and continued to stabilize. He'd earned the *Finding Nemo* theme on his incubator, reminding

us every day to "just keep swimming." On a daily basis, we would go to the NICU and read to him, help change his diaper, and just place our hands on his head and pray he would be healed. Crue knew when we were there, and we were determined to give him the best shot at a normal life.

That following Wednesday, we received a call from his primary nurse at 3:30 a.m. It was a call no mother of an NICU baby wants to receive. She told us they believed Crue had a bowel perforation and he needed to be transported to Children's Hospital. After transporting him, we waited for hours until they finally came back to get us so we could see our son. Crue was suffering from NEC, a condition that affects the bowel and is often fatal to preemies who are unable to fight off the infection. They informed us he was not responding to treatment. They also said his labs were falling and we needed to be prepared for him to die that day. Those words shook us to our core.

We went to his incubator, held his hand, and begged our son not to leave us. We told Crue we would fight for him if he would just hang on. We begged God not to take our son away from us. Crue was a fighter, and we needed him.

We knew our son was tired, so we made the decision to hold him for the first time and let him pass away in his mother's arms. We only wanted him to feel love. We told him how sorry we were for all his suffering. We told him how much we loved him and it was okay for him to go. Crue was surrounded by love when he gained those beautiful angel wings. He was so peaceful.

After losing Crue, we veered into a vulnerable state as a couple, which allowed us to fall even deeper in love with each other. We needed each other more than we could ever put into words, so we embraced that. As a mother who had just gone through all those traumatic events and being so sick herself, getting out of bed and seeing daylight was often too much to handle. The depression, anger, and isolation I felt was often suffocating. Having a husband who is also like a personal superhero to pick up all the broken pieces was a complete game changer. The patience we had shown to each other was one of the biggest aspects that allowed us to handle the incredible loss of our son and still stand stronger than ever afterward.

We definitely had our moments where we struggled through the loss, and we still do. The lasting effects of preeclampsia are daunting and extremely traumatic. We knew we wanted to try again for another baby, but because of the severity and the acuity of our delivery, we had to wait at least a year before our second attempt. We took that time to work on ourselves, both individually and as a couple. We found an amazing therapist who focused on loss and helped get our minds strong enough to go through another pregnancy again, but all while recognizing and dealing with the significant loss of our sweet Crue. As a couple, we had differing opinions regarding the timing of our next pregnancy, which caused a lot of stress. As a mother, it's easy to want to get pregnant quicker than the husband because you often feel it's the woman's body that "failed." It's easy to want to prove, together, we have the capability of bringing a healthy baby into this world. (We eventually welcomed a healthy baby boy in 2021.) Still to this day, we battle with the constant feeling our family will never be complete. A piece of our heart is in heaven.

Carrying the weight of that void continues to leave us in a state of panic, and we are often breathless when birthdays, holidays, and other milestones serve as the constant reminder our lives will never be the same.

Communication is such an important aspect of our relationship. We talk about everything: the good, bad, and the ugly. We talk out our emotions because it's so important to be able to feel the rawness of them and not bottle our feelings up inside. We often give each other space to grieve, but with the expectation we don't do it alone. We also started a nonprofit in honor of our son and our best friend's daughter, known as the Hayden and Crue Project, which helps serve the loss community and give back to those families who are going through the unthinkable. It has been a huge help for us while navigating our own loss. Grief is messy; it takes grace and patience with yourself, and your partner, during the unbearable days. Nothing in life can prepare you for losing a child. There are no regular discussions about pregnancy complications, nor is there a diagnosis that can prepare you for the consequences of losing your precious baby. There is no hurt like the one a mother and a father feel when their child passes away in their arms. Standing strong with one another and being that constant support during those unbearable days will help withstand any storm.

"I promise to find hope through the heartache; to find joy through the sadness; to find strength through the weakness; to love even when it's hard; to live freely and bravely even when I'm scared. To make the most of my days, to live in a way that would make you proud." –Author Unknown

For more information on our nonprofit, visit: www.TheHaydenandCrueProject.com

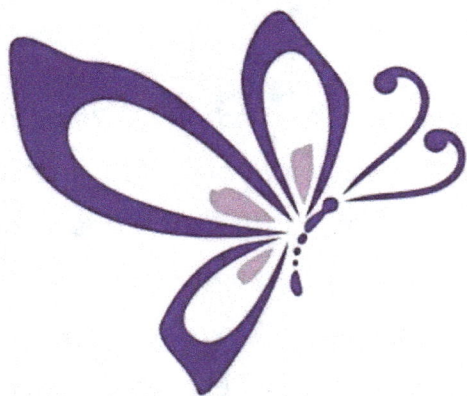

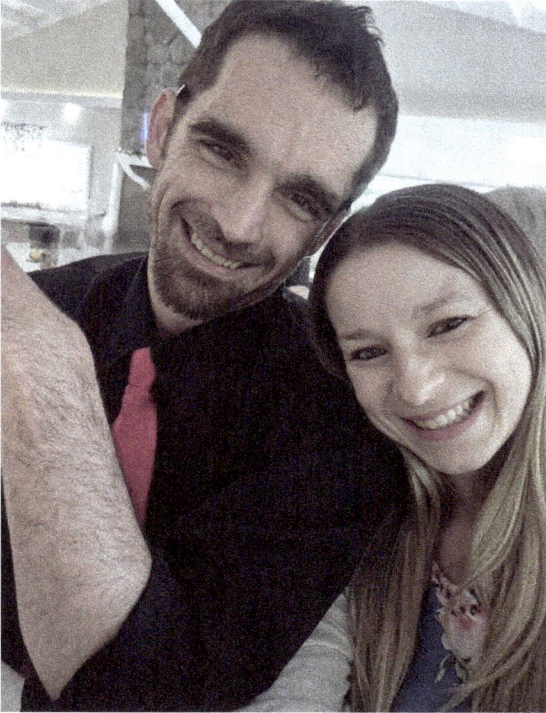

Ryan & Ashley Lehart

"Peanut:" Where their story began and ours continued.

We are a family of 4 living in Milford, Ohio. We have one dog. We love spending time as a family and enjoying all the moments together with our kids. We have one angel baby "Peanut", who will forever remind us to live life to the fullest.

It was December 6th, 2020, and I was looking at a positive pregnancy test. As the mother-to-be, I couldn't wait to share the news with my husband when he got home from work. I even made a card saying, *I can't wait to meet you, Daddy.* We both were thrilled with every emotion anyone could expect to have. However, little did we know we had just began a journey we never thought we would experience. Our baby quickly became known as "Peanut," and this is where their story began.

In January 2021, we scheduled our first appointment with the GYN because that is what the practice said we had to do first. We both continued to be excited over "Peanut" and enjoyed the easy pregnancy; there weren't really any symptoms. Looking back, maybe that was a sign we just didn't pick up. Christmas was quickly approaching, and we decided to share the news with our immediate families. We made a picture frame telling our parents they were going to be grandparents again. To this day, that is one of our favorite memories of "Peanut" because everyone got to experience the joy, until it was stripped away within a few short weeks.

January quickly came, and it was time for the first appointment, for which we both were very excited. The nurse practitioner confirmed we were, indeed, pregnant and had us schedule the first appointment with the OBGYN, which was the following week. COVID-19 restrictions were still in play, so both of us couldn't attend the appointment. As the mother attending by herself, I remember all the excitement I felt to see the other pregnant women in the waiting room. That appointment worried me, however, because the doctor said he couldn't hear the heartbeat on the doppler. Then, he said that was normally the case because I was only nine weeks pregnant. I remember going to work, praying everything would be fine. I continued to feel elated because "we were pregnant."

The following week, on January 20th, was the first ultrasound. That time, both of us were able to attend. We went to the ultrasound room and didn't know what to expect. After all, it was our first pregnancy. We both entered that room with so much excitement, but it was quickly taken away. The ultrasound technician was very nice, but we could just tell something was off. To this day, I remember saying, "That doesn't look like a baby." The sweet technician replied, "It's a baby, but there is no heartbeat." I don't know if she was supposed to tell us that or not, but we appreciated she did because we had a moment to prepare for what came next. They took us both to a room to wait for the doctor. The doctor came in after what felt like forever, but I'm sure it was only a few minutes. He was very kind and said he believed we were having a silent miscarriage but wanted to schedule another ultrasound the following week to confirm. We left that appointment feeling angry, sad, and confused. We did not believe what was going on. Even though our world seemed to stop, everything and everyone else kept going. We made the decision to tell our parents, our brothers, and our best friends about what had happened, which gave us additional support and help to navigate such a terrible thing. The next hours and days were nothing but a blur.

January 25th, 2021 came, and we went to the ultrasound, knowing it was going to prove what we already knew. In a way, we both hoped for a different outcome, for that ultrasound and "Peanut" to be just fine. We entered the appointment feeling numb, just wanting it to be over. That time, sitting in the waiting room with all the expectant mothers was not what we wanted to do. That ultrasound technician didn't seem to know why we were there. They said it was, "being a viability scan." After the scan was complete, we went back to the room to discuss options with the doctor because we were still pregnant. After a private discussion, the doctor returned, and we both opted for the D&C, which was scheduled for the next day.

Again, because of COVID-19 restrictions, both of us were not allowed in the hospital. We were alone, and that was an awful thing for both of us after we officially just lost our "Peanut."

The next several days all blended together with constant phone calls and condolences from others. However, we appreciated all the support we received from our family and friends. As a mother, I advocated for myself and reviewed the bereavement policy at work, which got me five days off to grieve in silence at home. Ryan returned to work the day following the D&C. We both grieved in our own ways and allowed one another to do so. We supported one another by allowing each other to talk about what we were feeling, as well as just being silent.

Losing "Peanut" impacted our relationship in many ways; it brought us closer together, as well as drove us a little further apart. We became closer because we had just experienced an awful tragedy. We grew a little further apart because we didn't know how to help one another. Navigating grief is challenging because it is different for everyone and we hadn't experienced grief like that before. It took us some time to fully discuss what we had just experienced, and it was hard seeing other people with kids because it made us wonder why it didn't work out for us. We focused on our love for one another, as well as faith we would find a purpose for "Peanut." Losing "Peanut" ultimately brought us closer together because, at the end of the day, we still had each other; that was everything.

We found comfort in talking about "Peanut" because we didn't want our first baby to be forgotten. Both of us made the difficult decision to share our loss and our grief online on social media because we didn't want to keep our experience hidden. We discovered miscarriage often leads to silent grief. It was really eye-opening when we shared our experience, to see how many other people experienced the same exact thing. The two of us began to advocate for "Peanut" and chose to share "Peanut's" memory with others. We decided if our terrible experience can help others going through the same thing, then that was "Peanut's purpose."

Moving forward was a challenge because both of us didn't know what we wanted our future to look like, nor did we really know what to expect or where to begin. There were days when our grief would come back, and it was like what we had experienced after that very first ultrasound. We were always told grief was like waves, as it can come crashing in at any time. To this day, that is very true. Being around pregnant women or families with kids is often a challenge. Yes, we are extremely happy for those families, but we are also very sad because we want those exact very things. We don't know if we will ever be able to experience them or have another positive pregnancy test. In fact, we never talked about when we would try for more kids because that just seemed like an impossible thing.

To this day, losing "Peanut" was the hardest thing we'd ever dealt with, both as a couple and individually. We grieved in our own ways but remained there for each other and helped one another navigate the grief. Truthfully, we might not ever fully process the loss of "Peanut," for many reasons we won't ever know. For anyone who is experiencing loss such as this, we want you to know how truly sorry we are, and we hope you might someday get your happy ending. It is okay to not be okay, as well as to cry or scream. Rely on each other and the love you each share; that good will help you through the dark times. Find comfort in knowing your sweet baby is loved, and will always be loved; nothing will change that or take that away from you. Your child mattered and made a difference. Do something every year to remember your baby. For us, it's "Peanut's" due date of August 12th. Each year, what we do looks a little different, but we take some time out of our busy day to remember "Peanut" and often wonder who they would have been. We choose to remember our "Peanut" each and every day. "Peanut" impacted us in many ways and allowed us to become stronger than ever.

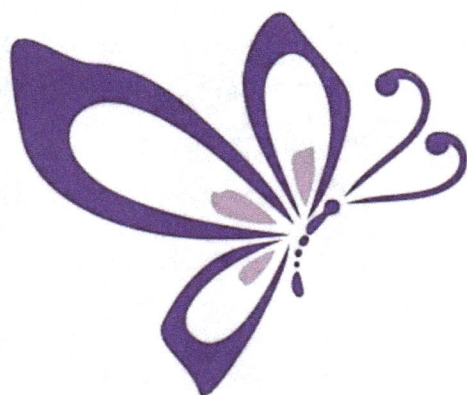

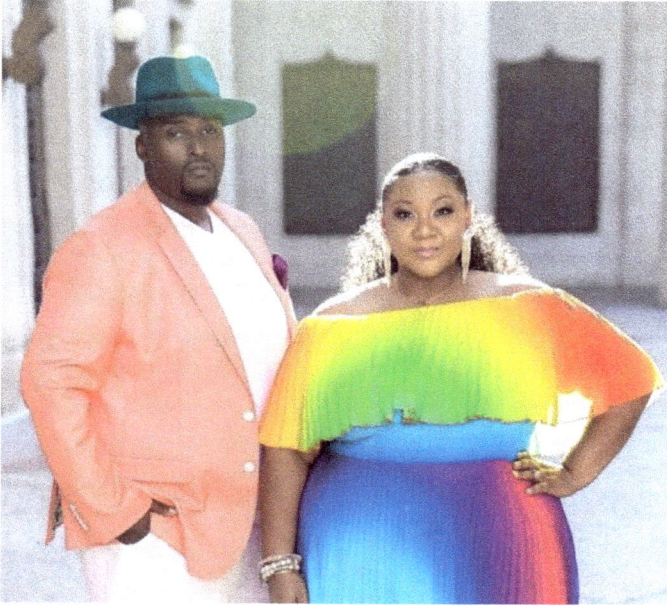

Marcus & Tondrea Maclin

Greetings from the Parents of Two Angels
and a Miracle!

Natives from Tennessee-Marcus from Memphis and Tondrea from Nashville. We took the big leap into our destiny and said "I do" to one another in 2011. We enjoy going to concerts, eating sushi, and keeping each other laughing. Our "road to Jeremiah" wasn't easy, but we hope our story encourages other couples to continue to pull together.

Our journey to where we are today has been long and challenging, filled with moments of deep sorrow and immense joy. Through it all, we've held on to our faith, which has carried us, even during our darkest hours.

We married in 2011, full of love and hope for the future. We prayed and asked the Lord for a year to travel and enjoy each other before starting a family. A little over a year into our marriage, we found out we were expecting. Little did we know what lay ahead. Our first pregnancy was filled with joy, but at sixteen weeks, concerns arose. A nurse practitioner's cold remark, "It's not looking so good," hit us hard. We kept holding on, clinging to each other and to our faith.

Life became a routine of appointments until the heartbreaking day on July 18, 2013, when we learned there was no heartbeat. Our stillborn daughter, Lyric Marche' Maclin, was delivered at twenty-six weeks on July 19, 2013. She was wrapped in a tiny handmade gown, and we held our beautiful baby girl for the first and the last time. Leaving the hospital that day was devastating, and we couldn't shake the feeling it was somehow our fault.

The loss of Lyric plunged us into deep grief. We turned to alcohol to numb the pain, but we realized we needed to find a healthier way to cope. We struggled to find support, often feeling like we were on an island, but we were thankful when God brought people into our lives who helped us begin to heal.

In 2017, we were thrilled to learn we were pregnant with our first son, Nehemiah James Maclin, nicknamed "Nehjay." That pregnancy felt different, and our first appointment was filled with joy. But soon after, things took a troubling turn. Nehemiah was growing slowly, and on December 26, 2017, Tondrea noticed bleeding. We rushed to the emergency room, fearing the worst. The hospital was eerily quiet, and we were taken to the maternity wing, where we learned Tondrea was in full-blown labor.

Nehemiah was born, but tragically, he did not survive.

Losing Nehemiah left us numb, filled with anger, embarrassment, and deep sorrow. We questioned everything again: *How can this happen to us a second time? What is wrong with us?* Once again, we were leaving the hospital empty-handed, overwhelmed with grief and despair.

We were lost, unsure about how to move forward. Anger, depression, guilt, regret, and disappointment hit us in waves. But once again, we knew we had to regroup and have that difficult conversation about grieving in a healthy way. The liquor store had become a familiar place, but we knew we couldn't keep turning to alcohol to numb our pain. We debated whether to share that part of our story, but we realized, without it, others wouldn't be able to fully understand the journey we've been on. Those eight years were incredibly hard, and we often found ourselves asking, *Why us?* again.

One night, while watching the movie *Sing* with a friend, we heard the words of "Hallelujah" by Leonard Cohen. Marcus was moved to tears, and during that moment, he heard the Lord say, "It's never easy being the example." It wasn't what we wanted to hear, but it was what we needed in order to begin healing. From that day forward, we looked for opportunities to be a blessing to others who had experienced loss.

In 2020, during the midst of the pandemic, the desire for a child never left our hearts. One day, Tondrea surprised Marcus with a positive pregnancy test. We cried together, overwhelmed by a mix of joy and fear. Our original OB assured us, "We are going to do everything we can to make sure you leave this hospital with a baby this time."

That pregnancy was filled with a mix of emotions: happiness, fear, and thankfulness. The doctors discovered Tondrea had a low S protein deficiency, which caused her placenta to clot during pregnancy. Knowing that was bittersweet. If we had known earlier, our previous pregnancies might have had different outcomes. However, we were overjoyed to learn there were steps we could take to prevent another loss. Tondrea began taking two Lovenox injections daily, and we told no one except our immediate families and a few trusted prayer warriors. We knew we had to be obedient and cautious.

Everything seemed to be going well, until one appointment, when the doctor noticed the blood flow in the placenta was reversing. They told us to go home, pack a bag, and prepare to be admitted until the baby was born. At just over twenty-three weeks, the prospect of staying in the hospital for months was daunting, but we trusted in the Lord. Marcus did everything he could to make that antepartum room feel like home.

Our OB visited us daily, monitoring the situation closely. As Thanksgiving approached, we were hopeful, but on November 27, 2020, just two hours after Marcus left for work, I called him back in tears. "The doctors said that Jeremiah is ready…" At only twenty-five weeks and five days, we were terrified, but we trusted God wouldn't leave us empty-handed that time. Marcus returned, we prayed together, and at 11:58 a.m., we welcomed our miracle boy, Jeremiah James Maclin, into the world. He weighed just one pound and five ounces.

The room was filled with worship as Jeremiah entered the world, and to everyone's surprise, he cried—a small but strong cry. Marcus's voice cracked with emotion as he asked, "Did my baby just cry?" The doctor smiled, replying, "He sure did, Dad."

Jeremiah spent ninety-three days in the NICU, defying all odds. He endured numerous trials, including an inguinal hernia that required surgery, but he came through it all stronger than ever. We were finally able to take him home on February 27, 2021. Today, Jeremiah is thriving, reaching milestones we could only dream of. He is our rainbow baby, a true miracle, and a testament to the power of faith, hope, and love.

Our journey to Jeremiah has been filled with challenges, heartache, and deep sorrow, but it has also been a journey of growth, healing, and unshakable faith. We are forever thankful for the lessons we've learned along the way and for the people who have walked the path with us. We hope our story can be a source of inspiration for others who are facing their own challenges. Never give up, hold on to hope, and trust in God's timing. He makes no mistakes.

Signed,

The Maclins

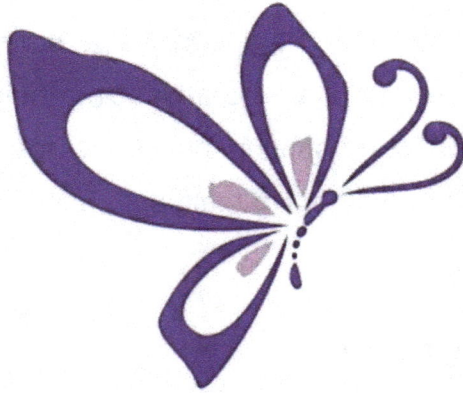

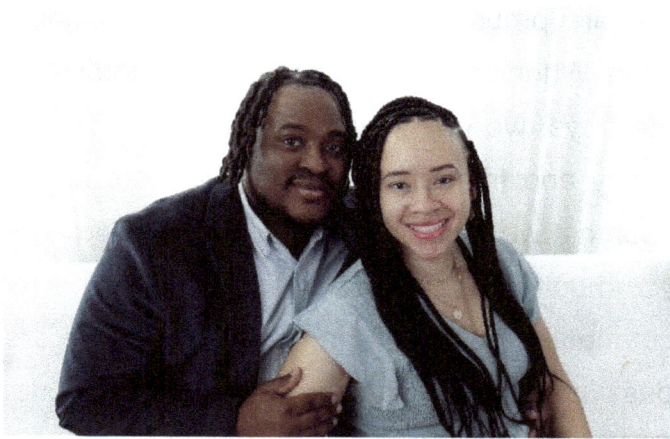

Antwon & Marquisse Watson

It's been said by Robert A. Heinlein, "Love is that condition in which the happiness of another person is essential to your own."

We are proud parents, residing in Cincinnati, Ohio. When we're not at a practice or game with the boys, we enjoy spending quality time with family and friends. As active members of our church, we are dedicated to serving our community and deepening our faith. As cofounders of The Alana Marie Project, we are passionate about effecting change in the world, especially within the pregnancy and infant loss community. Our shared commitment to faith, passion for making a difference, and love for new experiences bring us closer together each day.

The pure excitement of knowing we were bringing a life into this world together was second to none. We discovered so much joy with the different pregnancy apps and finding out the size of our baby as each week passed. As the weeks progressed, we finally made it to the twenty-week mark to find out Alana's gender.

An appointment which was supposed to be one of the best times of our lives turned out to be one of the most dreadful, heart-breaking moments we could have ever imagined during our young marriage. In addition to finding out we were having a baby girl, the doctor informed us Alana was behind on her growth and wasn't measuring out appropriately at that stage of the pregnancy. As a husband, it has always been my role to be optimistic and try to find some positivity through the tough news. My immediate thoughts were: *Maybe we aren't as far along as we thought*, and *Everything is okay*. But being a wife in the medical field, I knew things were not okay based on the questions coming from the tech.

We left that appointment full of uncertainty and fear but remained hopeful Alana would be okay. Little did we know, four weeks later, we would be giving birth because I was diagnosed with preeclampsia. That put Alana and I in immediate danger, and I had to be induced. The doctors said Alana had only a 10% chance of surviving the delivery. However, our precious girl defied the odds and not only survived the delivery but spent thirty-six amazing hours with us before she gained her heavenly wings.

During those living moments, we were able to love on her, pray over her, and share her with our friends and family. While that was not the ending, we were hoping and praying for, we found comfort in one another as we tried to navigate life together during that difficult time. We knew our new norm would include a rough journey ahead, but we also knew we would walk it out together through our faith, love, and support from our friends and family.

As we embraced this journey of grief, it opened up conversations with people sharing their stories of loss with us. We were astounded to find out so many people whom we knew had gone through a similar issue. That sparked a fire in us to create a healing environment of people just like us, a place that would allow people to share their journey and support others families in need. Out of our tragedy, we birthed The Alana Marie Project. The nonprofit focuses on encouraging, empowering, and supporting families who had lost a baby because of miscarriage, stillbirth, and infant death.

We have seen our organization reach families all over the US, and extend even as far as Japan. It has been a place for us to honor not only Alana's life, but so many other angel babies, as well. During that time, we have found healing in helping others heal. After the loss of our angel, Alana, we were blessed with three sons: AJ, Andrew, and Aiden.

At the beginning of 2024, we were excited about the idea of adding one more baby to the Watson family. Just when we thought we had a handle on this whole grief thing, we experienced not one, but two, miscarriages back-to-back ten years after losing Alana. The first miscarriage occurred in March 2024. We were about 5 weeks pregnant, when I started bleeding at home. We were very excited to find out we were pregnant again so soon after the first miscarriage. Unfortunately, we found out we were likely experiencing a second miscarriage during our ultrasound appointment, which was on Alana's tenth birthday. That was certainly not the way we dreamed of that appointment playing out. After getting a follow-up ultrasound two weeks later, it was confirmed that were indeed having a second miscarriage. After much discussion, we opted to have a D&C.

Our miscarriage journey has been tough. As this book is being written, we are freshly grieving the loss of two angel babies. While we are so extremely blessed to have three amazing sons in our lives, we were hopeful to close out our chapter by having a baby girl whom we could raise here on Earth. Unfortunately, our attempts have left us with heartache and pain. The toughest thing about the second miscarriage was finding out the baby was a girl, who went on to heaven to be with her big sister, Alana. There was something about knowing the gender of our baby that created a different kind of grief that was so unexpected. We could have never imagined the same community we created to support families grieving the loss of a baby would be a support for us! Many people whom we have connected with through this grief journey have been a support and encouragement as we grieve the two miscarriages we experienced.

The grief this time around had been much different than the loss of Alana. With Alana, the world experienced it with us. With the miscarriages, we experienced much of it alone because we hadn't shared with many people we were expecting either time. Unfortunately, we didn't have an opportunity to share the news with our parents, until we told them about the miscarriages.

When Alana passed away, we had no other children and could really take the time to grieve. After the miscarriages, it's been challenging to grieve in private away from our boys; we hadn't shared the news with them about either of the pregnancies. Despite the differences in how the grief looks for us this time around, a few things remain the same. First is our faith in God. We'd be lying if we said our faith hadn't been shaken, but we trust God will carry us through this, no matter how dark some of the days feel. Second, one thing we have learned throughout our grief journey is communication is essential. Intentional communication with one another has been so helpful for us. As hard as it can be, we strive to communicate regularly about how we are doing mentally and handling the grief. Third, leaning into support from family and friends has been so helpful as we navigate the new path of our grief journey. While the journey has been incredibly challenging, we are grateful for the love and support that surrounds us. We know we are not alone. With faith, communication, and the strength of our community, we will continue to find our way through. Thank you to our village for standing by us. You stepped in to care for our boys when we needed time to ourselves, offered us meals when we were too drained to cook, and simply listened without judgment when we needed to talk. You respected our space while also ensuring we knew we were not alone, reminding us that you were here to help in any way we needed. To other couples walking a similar path, we encourage you to lean into your village. Grief is heavy, and no one should carry it alone. Let your community support you, just as ours has supported us.

To learn more about The Alana Marie Project visit: https://thealanamarieproject.com/

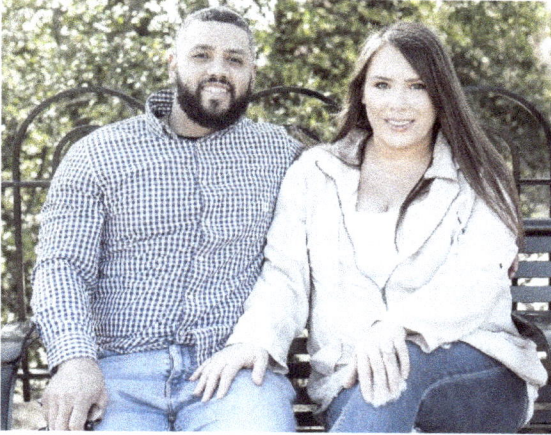

Curtis & Amanda Winkle

We believe in the transformative power of story. Everyone has a story, and that story drives their actions and their choices. Our stories lead us toward what we value most, and for us, that ultimate value is God.

We are a devoted couple with a blended family of five wonderful children. Our children range in age from 3 to 17. We have known each other since the age of 9 and have walked every stage of life together. This year we celebrate our 6th wedding anniversary.

This is our story. We were like most couples, just attempting to figure out life. We have known each other since we were nine years old. We grew up a few houses apart, attended the same schools, and were inseparable throughout our teenage years. We watched each other build lives and have babies with other people. We grew up together but carved separate paths for ourselves. Little did we know those paths would cross in the future and become intertwined into one life. Somewhere along the line, our friendship evolved, and we found ourselves making plans for a future. Still to this day, it's hard to comprehend how we got here.

After years of slowly developing our friendship into a relationship, we were ready for the next chapter. The beginning of the new chapter was swift. Within the same week, we had gotten married, bought a home, and united our girls as sisters. With a new home to fill, we realized the best way to complete our family dynamic was to have one final addition, a child we both shared biologically. In a world of his and hers, we were excited to have something that was "ours." The thought of our four daughters embarking on a united path to cultivate love, empathy, and joy into the new baby became a singular vison and passion for us. That pursuit was something which would alter the rest of our life.

Very shortly after, we found out we were expecting. It happened so quickly, and we both were thrilled. It felt as if our prayers had become our reality in the blink of an eye. We were living a dream we were so grateful for. Our lives were filled with victory after victory.

All nightmares begin as dreams. That fairy tale story unfortunately met its short-lived ending. We were sitting in an average hospital during a routine doctor's visit. It was the day when we would see our baby for the first time. We hadn't told the girls yet, and we were hoping for an ultrasound picture to share the news of their new baby brother or sister. Before we knew it, it was time to begin the ultrasound. Curtis was by Amanda's side, with one handing gripping hers and the other holding his phone, ready to record the moment. Curtis's eyes were glued to the black and white screen, and Amanda's scanned the nurse's expression. She was searching the nurse's face for anything that would give her some peace, waiting to hear the baby was perfect. Instead, the nurse's expressions changed. Not in an obvious way, but Amanda was studying her so intently she instantly knew. There was pause. The nurse looked up from the machine and asked Curtis to stop recording. He was taken back. Amanda's face lost much of her color. She repeated the nurses' instructions, "Curtis, please stop recording." Amanda looked over at his face, and her heart broke into a million pieces because she realized he was still blissfully unaware in just a moment their whole world would forever be different.

The nurse's next words were like a punch to the gut, like the winds that have gone far from a sail. We were deflated, confused, and speechless. "I cannot find the heartbeat; there is no heartbeat." Reality was slowly seeping in. Amanda's tears were cascading down her face like a window in a thunderstorm; she was looking at her husband for answers. The doctor walked in, with empathy dripping from her voice she explained what the next steps were, trying to process what that meant physically when the emotional weight was already more than we could bear. We left the facility completely broken.

Once home, it felt as if we walked in the door as new versions of ourselves. During our twenty years of knowing one another, that was the first time when we suddenly didn't know how to exist effortlessly in each other's presence. I kept thinking, *What do we talk about? If we talk about the baby, then we both get sad, but if we talk about anything else, it seems as if we're numb to what we just experienced.* We had to relearn what it was like to just be. The days of effortless conversation were at a standstill. We had to live in an uncomfortable stage where we didn't even know what to say to one another for a while.

Our processing of the miscarriage has not been an easy one. Unfortunately, denial played a large role. We vividly remember the games we would play in our heads to tell ourselves everything was going to be okay. We were convinced, after the D&C, life would revert back to normal and the pain would go away. That day came and went. The physical healing had gone smoothly, but the emotional pain was still very raw. At the time, we were waiting for the okay to start trying again. That day came and went, and to no surprise, it was not the magical healing we'd thought it would have been. We then moved on to thinking after we got pregnant again the pain would just be an awful memory. As beautiful of an experience it was briefly having our baby here, five years later, we are still weeping as we write this. The pain never goes away, as it shouldn't. We created a new life, and our children were getting a sibling. We discussed names and made plans, imagining how Christmas mornings would be forever changed, made even better. We were having a baby. And then, we weren't. The pain we wished away was the manifestation of our love for that sweet baby, suddenly gone. After all those years, we've learned to embrace that pain, to truly feel it. We felt it because we loved so deeply, because that baby was cherished, and wanted.

It's such a strange experience to lose our baby together but to grieve separately. Amanda was lost in a wasteland of pain and suffering. Curtis was lost in a tidal wave of obligations and solitude. If we could go back, we would do a million things differently. Grief feels like drowning, and yet we put the expectation on ourselves we were also supposed to save one another. If we were able to do it again, we'd give each other more grace. We'd also honor our sadness, and as weird as it sounds, we'd sit in it a little longer. We put a rush on our own healing, and the only thing we did was prolong it. We will mourn our baby until our last breath, but we made it on the other side of grief, and for that we are grateful.

Now being on the other side of that season of our lives, we can see the collateral beauty in what we went through. The Lord placed us in a furnace, and like clay at its final stage, He hardened our resilience, yet kept our hearts softened to His love. Those processes illuminated the oneness of our marriage and what it is capable of withstanding. The constant reminder of looking at your children and truly knowing what a gift they are. The beauty in truly leaning on God when your faith is being tested.

The beauty of experiencing every single moment with your baby that you thought was taken away from you forever. The experience of holding your rainbow baby for the first time, you are living the fulfillment of God's promise.

Life will bear many types of fruit; some sweet and nourishing, some bitter and sour. For us, we have found our solace in discovering the beauty during the time we spent in the desert. We leaned on our faith, and we grew in our relationship with God.

Psalm 77 has brought us comfort; that psalm reflects David's deep anguish and cry to God during a time of distress. David begins by expressing feelings of abandonment and questioning whether God has rejected him forever. He then recalls God's past faithfulness and wonders if God's promises and mercies have come to an end. Next, David shifts to remember God's mighty deeds in history, especially the Exodus, acknowledging God's ways are mysterious and beyond human understanding. David concludes with a reassertion of trust in God's power and a plea for God to act again in their present circumstances, knowing God's righteousness and strength endure forever.

Though that reflection, we found peace knowing the Lord has our baby but will not miscarry us.

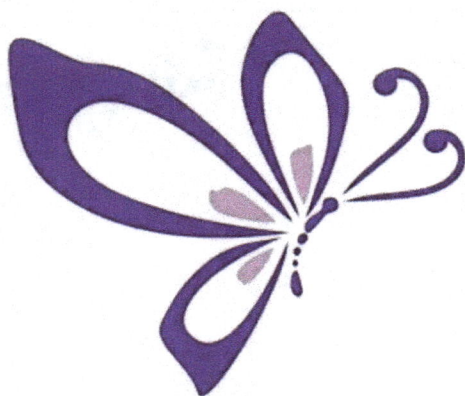

www.ingramcontent.com/pod-product-compliance
Lightning Source LLC
Chambersburg PA
CBHW052105270326
41931CB00012B/2891